# Carb Cycling:

# Carb Cycling Recipes

## *Simple And Delicious Carb Cycling Recipes For Rapid Fat Loss*

# Table Of Contents

Introduction......................................................................5

Chapter 1: Introduction to Carb Cycling.........................6

Chapter 2: The Carb Cycling Plans ...............................11

Chapter 3: Simple and Easy to Prepare Breakfast Recipes...........16

Easy Breakfast Omelet....................................................16

Healthy and Delicious Burrito.......................................18

Low-Carb Breakfast Tacos ............................................20

Delicious Breakfast Burrito ..........................................21

High-Carb Egg Muffin Special ......................................22

Your Favorite Breakfast Ham Omelet............................23

A Healthy BLT Sandwich...............................................25

Healthy Mini Egg Omelet..............................................26

Special Breakfast Enchilada..........................................28

Bacon-Wrapped Mini Meatloaf.....................................30

Low-Carb Egg Benedict Breakfast................................32

Avocado Grilled Chicken with Mango Salad.................34

Chapter 4: Simple and Delicious Lunch and Dinner Recipes ......36

3-Flavor Chicken ...........................................................36

Chicken Caribbean ........................................................38

Italian Chicken with Herbs ........................................................39

Lime Chicken with Spices ........................................................41

Baked Potatoes and Chicken ....................................................43

High-Carb Chicken and Turkey Medley......................................45

Pork Roast...............................................................................47

Healthy Baked Meatballs .........................................................49

Healthy BBQ............................................................................51

Delicious Turkey Burger...........................................................53

Healthy Steak Tenderloin.........................................................54

Roasted Beef with Stir-Fry Veggies ..........................................55

Low-Carb Blue Cheese Steak ...................................................57

Sirloin Steak with Veggies .......................................................59

Sweet Pork Tenderloin.............................................................61

Special Tenderloin with Herbs and Spices .................................63

Herbed Roast Pork with Garlic .................................................64

Grilled Chicken Wings..............................................................65

Low-Carb Meatballs Barbecue ..................................................66

Low-Carb Roasted Turkey.........................................................68

Delicious Salmon Fillet with Herbs and Spices ..........................70

Spicy Pork Tenderloin .............................................................72

Easy Garlic and Herb Shrimp Salad...........................................74

Perfect Salmon Fillet...............................................................75

Chapter 5: You can be Healthy ..........................................................77

Conclusion ..........................................................................................87

# Introduction

This book contains facts and interesting information about carb cycling and how it can help you lose weight.

*"Carb Cycling"* contains easy to prepare recipes that taste good, are high in nutritious value and prepared in accordance to the principles of carb cycling. Not your ordinary fad diet, carb cycling gives you the flexibility to choose the foods you want to eat, and provides dieters with the chance to indulge once a week. The recipes contained in this book are easy to understand, even first-time cooks can prepare them without encountering any difficulty.

The book gives you recipes for breakfast, lunch, and dinner so you have a variety of foods to choose from. It also contains important tips about losing weight and how you can take advantage of this easy-to-follow weight loss program.

Aside from the recipes, this book also has a list of the recommended daily allowance of regular foods.

Let's begin the journey.

# Chapter 1: Introduction to Carb Cycling

Those who have been trying to lose excess pounds are probably familiar with the more popular diet fads, diet craze and diet menu plans. These diet plans' popularity stems from their promise of helping users to lose weight fast. These plans have different concepts and attacks.

Among the most recognizable are the low-carb diet plans that promise people that they will receive immediate positive results. However, some of those who tried these types of diet plans reported gaining the weight they lost right after reintroducing carbohydrates into their diets.

From popular trainer and transformation specialist, Chris Powell, comes carb cycling, a diet plan that alternates high-carb and low-carb days. How is it different from all the other weight loss plans before it?

*What is it exactly?*

It's a simple diet plan that takes advantage of the benefits of reduced carbohydrate and increased carbohydrate techniques. This plan has reward days or meals, allowing you to still eat your favorites even if you're on a diet. Unlike other diet plans that restrict and completely change your eating habits, this plan does not make you feel "food-deprived". If you follow this plan, then you can still eat foods that are healthy and enjoy the foods you love, but still get rid of those excess pounds. Is it too good to be true?

*The Basics*

The plan allows users to go from a low-carb day to a high-carb day and a reward day each week, but it still follows some of the basics in losing weight:

- You are allowed to eat five small meals a day.

- You have to eat breakfast not later than 30 minutes after waking up. Your high-carb meal should include protein and carbohydrates.

- Succeeding meals after breakfast should have a 3-hour interval.

- The meals should include only those "approved foods".

- Consume at least 1 gallon of water or allow fluids.

*How Carb Cycling Works*

For you to shed off some unwanted weight, your body would need a combination of carbohydrates, proteins and fats.

- *Carbohydrates* – Carbohydrates are your body's number 1 source of fuel. You can get the carbs you need from healthy sources like fruits, vegetables, legumes and grains. Take note of the unhealthy sources of carbohydrates; some of which are cookies, cakes, doughnuts, soda, candies and processed foods. Good carbohydrates are essential for your body's ability to burn calories because they are slowly broken down by the digestive tract than those unhealthy ones. These healthy carbohydrates ensure that your body's blood sugar is kept at acceptable levels while your energy levels remain steady.

- *Proteins* – They help build and maintain muscle mass. These muscles are important in burning fat. Proteins break down more slowly than carbohydrates and fat, thus burning more calories and keep you feeling full longer.

- *Healthy fats* – These are unsaturated fats that should still be included in your diet but intake should be controlled and properly monitored. They help in the development and the proper function of your brain and eyes. They help reduce the risks of developing heart conditions and depression and prevent arthritis. They also help manage your body's energy levels and curb your appetite.

What's the principle behind alternating low-carb and high-carb days? You see, during a high-carb day, your body stocks up so that when you are on a low-carb day, you still burn unwanted fats. This actually works well with your metabolism so that your body burns more calories even during the days when you have to eat low-carb meals.

Eating more every other day and cutting down on the days in between is an effective way of intensifying the weight loss process while still efficiently maintaining your fat-burning muscles. This is a diet plan that you can use for short-term and long-term weight loss.

*What Happens*

Eating breakfast not later than 30 minutes after you wake up jumpstarts your body's metabolism. It also ensures that you have the fuel you need for the whole day. During your high-carb days, having your meals at three-hour intervals boosts your metabolism, provides fuel for your muscles and organs and delivers the vitamins and fibers the body needs.

On low-carb days, you burn the fat while maintaining your muscles. It also helps balance your hormones and delivers the needed vitamins and fibers to your body.

During your reward days, you reset your system so it is ready for another cycle. It helps satisfy your cravings so you don't feel deprived while losing weight. At the same time, you are rewarding yourself for your progress. It also jacks up your calorie-intake but ensures that it is limited to maintenance level. It also boosts your metabolism while developing the calorie-burning muscles.

*How to Keep it Going*

It would be beneficial to restart your carb-cycling engine. While this plan prevents your body from reaching a plateau, your body will eventually "understand" the process and soon your metabolism drops which will result in the slowing down of the weight loss process. In order to re-fire, you need to devote one whole week each month to eating high-carb diet only. This means that you'll be eating normally like your high-carb days. By the end of the week, your metabolism gets a big boost and it is ready to burn those calories again. This is referred to as the Slingshot technique.

What are the benefits that can be derived from carb cycling?

- This plan fits in any kind of lifestyle.

- You will learn the basic principles of losing weight and maintaining your ideal weight.

- You can have control over your life, not just on losing weight.

- You remain active and energy levels are always up.

- You can still eat your favorite foods.

- It helps you to build leaner and stronger muscles.

- Empowerment, physically, emotionally, mentally and spiritually.

# Chapter 2: The Carb Cycling Plans

This section will briefly discuss the different diet plans. It is important that you know this before giving you the recipes to try.

*The Easy Cycle*

The Easy Cycle is for those who cannot afford not to eat their favorite foods but would still want to lose weight. This cycle lets you alternate on low-carb and high-carb days; and on each single high-carb day, you can eat your reward meal, as long as you don't consume it for dinner. So, with the Easy Cycle, you can still enjoy your favorite foods, four days a week and still lose the amount of weight you intend to lose.

This cycle allows you to satisfy your favorite food cravings during your low-carb days.

*How does it work?*

You will have to follow a low-carb/high-carb diet for your non-reward meals. While you can still reward yourself, you'll only do so less often. For instance, you usually consume 7 servings of ice cream each week. Following the Easy Cycle plan, you will be only consuming 4 bowls per week. So, you still get to eat your favorite sweet dessert and you still lose weight.

*Your Week at a Glance*

>   Monday – Low-Carb

>   Tuesday – High-Carb plus One Reward Meal

Wednesday – Low-Carb

Thursday – High-Carb plus One Reward Meal

Friday – Low-Carb

Saturday – High-Carb plus One Reward Meal

Sunday – High-Carb plus One Reward Meal

For all your meals, either for high-carb or low-carb day, it is better to eat smaller portions. The more calories you cut, the more weight you lose.

On the other hand, the weight loss with the Easy Cycle plan is not as fast as the other cycles. This plan is a workable plan when you are just starting to change your eating habits. You can easily switch to other plans should you decide to do so.

*Classic Carb Cycle*

The Classic Carb Cycle is the simplest plan out of the 4. It makes you lose weight faster and helps you to maintain your ideal weight.

*Your Week at a Glance*

Monday – Low-Carb

Tuesday – High-Carb

Wednesday – Low-Carb

Thursday – High-Carb

Friday – Low-Carb

Saturday – High-Carb

Sunday – Reward Day

*Turbo Carb Cycle*

From the name itself, you'll know that this plan allows you to lose more extra pounds faster. You will notice that the low-carb days come after the other so you burn fats two days in a row, allowing you to lose weight quicker.

*Your Week at a Glance*

Monday – Low-Carb

Tuesday – Low-Carb

Wednesday – High-Carb

Thursday – Low Carb

Friday – Low-Carb

Saturday – High-Carb

Sunday – Reward Day

*Fit Carb Cycle*

The Fit Carb Cycle allows you to get lean muscles without sacrificing your athletic performance. This plan eliminates fat and supplies fuel to your body to help you perform successfully, whatever sport you engage in. Notice there are 2 consecutive days for high-carb because it allows your muscles to absorb more fuel, which you'll need for maximum sports performance.

When you need to go low-carb, your body's glucose supply becomes depleted and your muscles become more sensitive to insulin. So, when you have a high-carb or a reward day, your muscles will absorb more carbohydrates, allowing you to burn extra fuel instead of storing it as fat.

*Your Week at a Glance*

> Monday – High-Carb
>
> Tuesday – High-Carb
>
> Wednesday – Low-Carb
>
> Thursday – High-Carb
>
> Friday – High-Carb
>
> Saturday – Low-Carb
>
> Sunday – Reward Day

You can alternately follow the different cycles if it works for you.


*Getting Started*

If you have a strong desire to transform your body and your life, this helps you get started.

1. Choose a promise

   This can be considered as the most important part of your weight loss journey. You begin by setting a goal (or a promise) that you will have to keep. Make specific and doable (realistic) goals (promises). There is no point in setting your goals when you cannot achieve them. This will be your guide as you go along your weight loss journey.

2. Choose an eating plan

   Decide based on the information that you read above. Choose one which you are confident that you can do without fail. You can begin with the Easy Cycle because it's the easiest among the 4 eating plans. You can easily switch to a plan when you think you are ready; carb cycling is that flexible.

The good thing about carb cycling is that it also prevents you from reaching a plateau. Most dieters, when they have been constantly losing weight, usually hit a plateau wherein their weight loss stops even without changing their diet plan. With carb cycling, you don't have to worry about it. The beauty of this weight loss plan is that you are given choices and you are not forced to follow something that you have difficulty doing.

Now that you have learned some of the basics of this unique menu diet plan, you are now ready to learn some recipes that you can incorporate in your diet. Your journey to losing weight and transforming your life starts now.

# Chapter 3: Simple and Easy to Prepare Breakfast Recipes

The principle for carb cycling is simple, there are days when you eat more carbs and days when you eat less of them, plus you get a reward day (depending on the type of eating plan you choose). It is easy and doable, that's why more and more people are switching to this weight loss plan.

This book will give you recipe ideas to help you in your journey to losing weight via carb cycling.

### *Easy Breakfast Omelet*

This is a great and healthy way to start your day. Eggs are among the richest sources of protein and these are inexpensive, too. Make a high-carb breakfast by mixing in fruits, whole grain toast, or oatmeal. You can prepare this for lunch or dinner and change the ratios depending on whether you are on a high-carb or low-carb day.

*Ingredients:*

- 4 egg whites

- 1 medium onion, chopped

- 1 medium bell pepper, chopped

- Mushrooms, chopped

- 1 medium tomato, chopped

- Spinach

- Olive oil in spray bottle

- A dash of salt and pepper or low –sodium seasoning blend

*Note:* You can make use of any other filling that you like. This makes 1 serving, if you want more, double the portions accordingly.

*Procedure:*

1. In a small bowl, whisk the egg whites for at least 45 seconds.

2. Add the vegetables and mix.

3. Spray olive oil on a non-stick pan and set to medium to high heat.

4. Add the egg whites and the veggie mixture into the pan. Season.

5. Let the omelet to finish cooking on one side and flip over to the other side with a spatula, to let it cook.

### Healthy and Delicious Burrito

*Ingredients:*

- 6 egg whites

- 4 tbsp ground turkey

- 2 handfuls spinach

- 2-4 leaves romaine lettuce

- 2 tbsp salsa

- Vegetable oil in spray bottle

- A dash of salt and pepper

*Note:* This makes 2 servings, double the recipe if you want more.

*Procedure:*

1. Spray oil in a non-stick pan and set to medium heat.

2. Cook turkey in oil. Set aside.

3. In a large mixing bowl, beat egg whites.

4. Using another non-stick pan, spray vegetable oil and set to medium to high heat. Cook the egg in the pan. As the egg begins to set, add in the turkey and spinach. Season. Let it cook further.

5. When cooked, wrap the turkey, egg and spinach combo in two or four leaves of romaine lettuce.

6. Garnish with the salsa and roll it up.

## Low-Carb Breakfast Tacos

*Ingredients:*

- 4 egg whites
- Corn tortillas
- 3 tomatoes, sliced
- 3 tbsp salsa
- A dash of low-sodium spice blend
- Oil in spray bottle

*Note:* This recipe makes 1 serving, double if you want to or adjust ingredients according to what you need.

*Procedure:*

1. Spray oil onto a non-stick pan. Set to medium heat.
2. Whisk the egg whites.
3. Season with the spice blend.
4. Cook until you get your preferred "scrambled" consistency.
5. Serve with corn tortillas.
6. Add in salsa and tomato slices.

## Delicious Breakfast Burrito

*Ingredients:*

- 1 tsp canola oil

- ¼ cup onions, chopped

- 2 egg whites, whisked

- 1 low-carb high fiber tortilla

- A pinch of salt

- A pinch of pepper

- Salsa

*Note:* This makes 1 serving of breakfast burrito. Adjust portions accordingly.

*Procedure:*

1. Set a non-stick pan to medium heat and cook the onions until soft.

2. Season with salt and pepper.

3. Add in beaten egg whites. Cook until almost set. Set aside.

4. Warm tortilla in a dry pan. Pour in cooked eggs on top of the tortilla and add salsa.

5. Roll up and eat.

### High-Carb Egg Muffin Special

*Ingredients:*

- 8 egg whites

- 4 slices of tomatoes

- 2 toasted English muffins

- A dash of low-sodium spice blend

*Note:* This recipe is good for a double-serving, add portions accordingly if you want to make more.

*Procedure:*

1. Whisk egg whites in a mixing bowl.

2. Spray oil in a non-stick pan. Set over medium to high heat.

3. Add the beaten eggs to the pan. Cook.

4. Add the sliced tomatoes and cooked eggs on the toasted muffin.

5. Season.

## Your Favorite Breakfast Ham Omelet

*Ingredients:*

- 3 egg whites, whisked
- 2 tbsp low-sodium ham, chopped
- 1 tbsp onions, chopped
- 1 tbsp green bell pepper, chopped
- 1 tbsp tomato, sliced
- Fresh salsa
- A portion of cheddar cheese
- A dash of salt and pepper or low-sodium spice blend

*Note:* This makes 1 serving, you can double the portions if you want to make it for two persons.

*Procedure:*

1. Heat a non-stick pan to medium-high.
2. Add the beaten egg whites. Season.
3. Let the egg whites set on one side.
4. Place the ham, onions, bell peppers and tomatoes in the middle and continue cooking. Fold in half to enclose filling.

5. Add salsa and cheese before serving.

## A Healthy BLT Sandwich

This is perfect for an anytime of the day meal as it is easy to prepare. It's ready in minutes so if you are late for work or an appointment, this will be great to perk up your day.

*Ingredients:*

- 2 wheat bread slices, toasted

- 2 medium tomatoes, sliced

- 2oz lean turkey breast

- 2 turkey bacon, cooked

- 2 green lettuce leaves

*Note:* This recipe is good for one, adjust accordingly.

*Procedure:*

1. Simply layer the meats, tomato slices, and lettuce between the toast and you're good to go.

### Healthy Mini Egg Omelet

*Ingredients:*

- 4 cups broccoli
- 4 whole eggs
- 1 cup egg whites
- ¼ cup low-fat cheddar cheese, shredded
- ¼ cup pecorino Romano cheese, shredded
- Salt and pepper to taste
- Cooking spray

*Note:* This recipe makes 4 mini omelets. Double the portions if you need more.

*Procedure:*

1. Preheat oven to 350°.

2. Steam the broccoli in water for 6 to 7 minutes. When cooked, crush into smaller pieces.

3. Add olive oil and season with salt and pepper.

4. Spray a standard non-stick cupcake molder with cooking spray and put broccoli mixture evenly into 9 molds.

5. In a mixing bowl, beat whole eggs, egg whites and grated pecorino Romano cheese. Add salt and pepper to taste. Pour over the broccoli mixture until mold is ¾ full.

6. Top each with grated cheddar cheese.

7. Bake for at least 20 minutes.

8. Serve immediately. If you have leftovers, wrap them in plastic wrap or put in a zip-lock plastic bag and refrigerate. It is good for one week.

## Special Breakfast Enchilada

*Ingredients:*

- 3 cups egg whites  (from about 18 large eggs)

- 2 tbsp water

- Salt and pepper to taste

- Cooking spray

- 1 tsp olive oil

- ½ cup chopped scallions

- 1 medium diced tomatoes

- 2 tbsp chopped cilantro

- 10 oz pack frozen spinach

- 4.5 oz can chopped green chilis

- Salt and pepper to taste

- ½ cup grated cheese

- 1 cup green enchilada sauce

- 1 medium avocado, diced

*Note:* This recipe yields 6 servings.

*Procedure:*

1. Preheat oven to350°F.

2. Pour in 1/ cup enchilada sauce on the bottom of a baking dish (9x12 inches).

3. In a mixing bowl, beat egg whites, add water, and a pinch of salt and pepper.

4. Coat a non-stick pan with cooking spray and set stove to medium heat.

5. Add ½ cup of the egg whites, swirl evenly to cover the entire pan. Cook for about 2 minutes and then flip to cook the other side. Set aside and repeat with the remaining egg whites. You should be able to make 6 "egg tortillas".

6. Heat oil in another non-stick pan and set to medium heat. Cook the scallions for about 2 to 3 minutes. Add tomato and cilantro. Add salt and pepper to taste and cook for another 1 minute. Add in spinach and green chili and let it cook for another 5 minutes. Adjust seasoning according to your preference.

7. Remove from heat and add ½ cup of cheese and mix well.

8. Divide spinach among the "egg tortillas". Roll up and place each side down in the baking dish. Top the "tortillas" with your remaining enchilada sauce and cheese. Cover the baking dish with foil and bake until cheese is melted, which will take about 20 to 25 minutes.

9. You can serve topped with diced scallions and avocados.

## Bacon-Wrapped Mini Meatloaf

*Ingredients:*

- 1 lb lean ground beef

- ½ lb bacon, cut in chunks

- 8 strips of bacon (do not cut)

- ¼ cup coconut milk

- 2 cloves minced garlic

- ½ cup minced fresh chives

- Chopped, fresh parsley

- Ground black pepper

*Note:* This recipe serves 4 people.

*Procedure:*

1. Preheat oven to 400°F.

2. In a mixing bowl, mix ground beef, bacon chunks, garlic, chives, and coconut milk. Season with ground black pepper. Bacon replaces salt.

3. Put one bacon slice each on a medium-sized muffin molder, creating rings.

4. Fill the rings with the mixed beef.

5. Cook in the oven for about 30 minutes.

6. Remove the mini meatloaf and top with parsley.

7. This is a good low-carb day breakfast.

## Low-Carb Egg Benedict Breakfast

*Ingredients:*

- 2 tbsp butter

- 1 beaten egg

- 1 slice ham

- Lazy hollandaise sauce

*For Hollandaise Sauce*

- ¼ cup mayonnaise

- 1 tsp lemon or lime juice

- ¼ tsp pepper

*Note:* This recipe is good for one; adjust if serving 2 or more.

*Procedure:*

1. In a small non-stick skillet, heat butter and add egg. Allow the egg to form into a solid mass; if you have an "egg ring", it is perfect for this. Flip to cook the other side.

2. Let the egg cool for about 2 to 3 minutes.

3. With the use of a regular drinking glass or a circle cookie cutter, cut the ham to fit the scrambled eggs' diameter. You

might need to fold the cooked egg several times to create a layer.

4. Cut the cooked egg to look like a muffin and place on top of the ham.

5. Top with hollandaise sauce.

*How to Make Hollandaise Sauce*

1. Blend all the ingredients for the sauce. Heat before topping onto your egg Benedict.

## Avocado Grilled Chicken with Mango Salad

*Ingredients:*

- 1 lb chicken breast

- 1 cup avocado, diced

- 1 cup mango, diced (1 ½ mangoes)

- 2 tbsp red onion, diced

- 6 cups baby red lettuce

*For the Vinaigrette*

- 2 tbsp olive oil

- 2 tbsp balsamic vinegar

- Salt and pepper

-

*Procedure:*

1. Grill chicken breasts and slice lengthwise. Put in a salad bowl.

2. Whisk together the ingredients for the vinaigrette and set aside.

3. Toss avocado, mango, red onion and sliced chicken breasts.

4. Line a salad platter with the baby lettuce and place the avocado and chicken mixture.

5. Drizzle with the vinaigrette just before serving.

6. This low-carb chicken salad is not just perfect for breakfast but also for lunch and dinner.

# Chapter 4: Simple and Delicious Lunch and Dinner Recipes

These recipes are easy, simple and delicious; plus they all have the right ingredients to ensure that you are on the right track.

### *3-Flavor Chicken*

*Ingredients:*

- 2 chicken breasts

- Olive oil in a spray bottle

- Baby spinach leaves, blanched

- 1 medium tomato, sliced

- 2 tsp each of tomato, basil, and garlic seasoning

*Note:* This recipe makes 2 portions; you can double the ingredients to make 4, and so on.

*Procedure:*

1. Season chicken breasts on both sides.

2. Set a non-stick pan to medium heat and spray olive oil.

3. Add the seasoned chicken breasts and cook on each side.

4. Serve with tomatoes and spinach. You may also sprinkle some oil or seasoning on the veggies.

5. Another option is to season with balsamic vinegar.

## Chicken Caribbean

*Ingredients:*

- 2 chicken breasts (skinless)

- Olive oil in a spray bottle

- 1 tsp low sodium soy sauce

- 1 tsp cider vinegar

- 1 tbsp Caribbean jerk seasoning

- 1 tsp water

*Note:* This makes 2 servings, adjust accordingly if you want to make more.

*Procedure:*

1. In a zip-lock bag or a container with cover, place all the ingredients. Massage the chicken gently until it is fully coated with marinade.

2. Let the marinated chicken sit for at least 30 to 45 minutes.

3. Grill the chicken over medium oil. You can also broil if you want to.

4. Serve hot with your veggie salad for low-carb days or brown rice for high-carb days.

For more flavorful chicken, you can marinate overnight. You may also keep it in the refrigerator (if you are making a batch) and cook when needed.

## Italian Chicken with Herbs

*Ingredients:*

- 2 chicken breasts, boneless and skinless

- Olive in spray bottle

- A dash of dried red pepper, ground

- 1/3 tsp salt

- ½ tsp Italian seasoning

- 4 tsp red wine vinegar

- 1 tsp water

*Note:* This recipe makes 2 portions, double the measurements if you are preparing more.

*Procedure:*

1. In a zip-lock bag (you can also use a container with cover), place all the ingredients. Make sure the chicken is coated with the marinade. Leave for at least 30 minutes. To make it more flavorful, prepare the day before you intend to cook it and just keep in the refrigerator.

2. Grill chicken over medium to high heat, cooking on each side.

3.  For a low-carb day, add in your favorite vegetable salad. You can also drizzle the chicken with a few drops of salad dressing.

4.  For high-carb days, serve with brown rice and a side dish of steamed                                                            veggies.

## Lime Chicken with Spices

*Ingredients:*

- 2 chicken breast halves, boneless and skinless
- 2 tsp butter
- 2 tsp olive oil
- 2 tbsp low sodium chicken broth
- 1 ½ tbsp lime juice
- ¼ tsp salt
- ¼ tsp pepper
- ½ tsp garlic powder
- ¼ tsp onion powder
- A pinch of cayenne pepper
- A pinch of paprika
- ¼ tsp thyme

*Note:* This is good for 2; adjust portioning when you intend to serve more.

*Procedure:*

1.  Mix together the seasonings and the chicken breast in a large zip-lock bag. Make sure that the chicken is well-coated. Let it stand for at least 1 hour to let the flavor set in. If you want to make it more flavorful, marinate the chicken overnight.

2.  Set a non-stick skillet to medium heat and put the butter and olive oil.

3.  When butter is melted, add in the chicken breasts and cook on each side.

4.  Remove from pan and set aside.

5.  To the same skillet, add the lime juice and the chicken broth. With the use of a whisk, mix the liquids and continue boiling until sauce is slight reduced.

6.  Add the cooked chicken into the skillet and coat with the sauce.

7.  Serve with blanched asparagus or broccoli on low-carb days. On the other hand, serve with sweet potatoes on your high-carb days.

8.  You may add grated cheese on reward days.

## Baked Potatoes and Chicken

This is a complete meal that the whole family will love, whether or not they are also on a diet.

*Ingredients:*

- 2 chicken breasts, skinless, diced

- 1 lb red potatoes

- Oil in spray bottle

- A bunch of asparagus, trimmed and cut into 1-inch pieces (you can also use red and green bell pepper or any other vegetable you like)

- 1/3 fresh basil, chopped

- 4 gloves of garlic, thinly sliced

- 1 ½ tbsp olive oil

- 1 tsp fresh rosemary, chopped

- A pinch of ground pepper to taste

- ½ cup chicken broth (optional)

*Note:* This is good for one person only but if you have to prepare for more people, you can adjust measurement accordingly.

*Procedure:*

1. Preheat oven to 400°.

2. Spray your baking dish with oil and place the chicken breasts, potatoes, tomatoes, vegetables, basil, garlic, olive oil and chicken broth. Sprinkle fresh rosemary and ground pepper.

3. Bake for about 45 minutes, checking and turning occasionally to make sure both sides are cooked.

4. Serve.

### High-Carb Chicken and Turkey Medley

*Ingredients:*

- 2 chicken breasts, boneless and skinless
- 2 slices Turkey bacon slices, diced
- Olive oil in spray bottle
- 1 ½ tsp butter
- ¼ cup apple, diced
- 2 ½ tbsp apple cider
- 1 cup brown rice
- 2 ½ tbsp low-sodium chicken broth
- 1 tsp thyme, dried
- salt and pepper

*Note:* This recipe serves only 1 person, adjust measurements if preparing for more than 1.

*Procedure:*

1. Spray oil on a non-stick pan and set to medium heat.

2. Put the chicken breasts to the pan and season with salt and pepper. Cook both sides.

3. Remove cooked chicken from pan and set aside.

4. In the same pan, cook the turkey bacon for about 5 minutes or until it turns brown.

5. Add apple and thyme. Add another pinch of salt and pepper.

6. When the apples turn to brown, bring in the apple cider and chicken broth.

7. Increase to high heat.

8. Let the sauce cook until it thickens, don't forget to stir continuously.

9. Add in butter and let it melt.

10. Next, put back in the pan and coat with the sauce. Simmer for about 2 to 3 minutes.

11. You can serve with brown rice.

12. If you making several batches, you can store in the freezer and simply reheat when needed.

## *Pork Roast*

*Ingredients:*

- 1 lb pork tenderloin

- 5 gloves of garlic, minced

- 1 tsp dried parsley flakes

- ½ tsp dried thyme leaves

- 1 tsp pepper

- 1 tbsp lemon juice (you can also use lime juice, depending on what's available)

- 1 tsp olive oil

*Note:* This recipe can serve at least 4 people.


*Procedure:*

1. Preheat oven at 450°F.

2. Line a roasting pan with foil and spray with oil.

3. In a mixing bowl, combine garlic, parsley, thyme and pepper.

4. In a small cup, put the lemon juice.

5. Brush pork with lemon juice and then rub with the garlic and spice mixture over the top and both its sides. Place in the roasting pan with the garlic and spice marinade side up.

6. Bake for about 35 minutes or until pork is evenly cooked.

7. Let the pork stand for 5 to 10 minutes before cutting and serving.

8. Serve with your favorite vegetable salad.

### Healthy Baked Meatballs

*Ingredients:*

- 16oz ground Turkey meat (93% lean)

- 2 egg whites

- 1/2  cup oatmeal

- ¼ cup nonfat milk

- ½ cup parsley

- 1 tbsp onions, dehydrated flakes

- ½ tsp oregano, ground

- ½ tsp garlic powder

*Note:* This recipe serves 4 with about 8 meatballs each.

*Procedure:*

1. Preheat oven at 400°F.

2. Spray a baking dish with oil.

3. In a mixing bowl, combine egg whites, oats and milk. Add in parsley, oregano, onions, garlic power and mix well. Add in ground turkey and mix well.

4. Make about 32 uniform meatballs (about 1 scoop).

5. Line in the baking dish, with a good distance from one another.

6. Bake in the oven for about 7 to 10 minutes or until the inside is cooked.

7. Serve with brown rice for high-carb days or vegetable salad on low-carb days.

## Healthy BBQ

*Ingredients:*

- 1 ¼ lbs boneless pork tenderloin, lean

- Sea salt

- Ground black pepper

- Garlic powder

- ¼ cup and 2 tbsp barbecue sauce (separate)

- Olive oil spray

*Note:* This BBQ recipe yields 4 servings.

*Procedure:*

1. Slice pork tenderloin in half, crosswise, and then slice each half lengthwise into quarters, yielding 8 strips. Season slices with sea salt, ground pepper and garlic powder. Place pork in a zip-lock plastic bag. Spoon ¼ cup of BBQ sauce and mix with the pork. Refrigerate overnight.

2. Pre-heat broiler. Line a baking sheet with aluminum foil and lightly spray with oil.

3. Place strips on the baking sheet in a single layer.

4. Broil for 2 to 3 minutes. Flip on the other side and continue to broil for 2 to 3 minutes more.

5. Serve with the sauce dripping. Serve with brown rice for high-carb days and vegetable salad with light dressing on low-carb days.

## Delicious Turkey Burger

*Ingredients:*

- 8 oz raw ground turkey

- Olive oil in a spray bottle

- 1 tsp minced garlic

- ¼ tsp cayenne pepper

- ½ tsp hot sauce (optional)

*Note:* This recipe serves two persons; you can adjust measurements as needed.

*Procedure:*

1. In a mixing bowl, combine the ground turkey with cayenne pepper and garlic. Add in the hot sauce if you want. Make sure the turkey and the seasonings are mixed thoroughly. Form into patties.

2. Spray oil in a non-stick pan and set to medium heat. Cook turkey patties on each side.

3. Serve immediately with carrot and celery sticks for low-carb days and boiled red potatoes on high-carb days.

### Healthy Steak Tenderloin

*Ingredients:*

- 6 oz sirloin steak, lean and boneless

- Olive oil in spray bottle

- ¾ steak seasoning

- 1 tsp parsley flakes

- 1 tsp rosemary flakes

*Note:* This recipe makes 2 servings, you may add portions if you need more.

*Procedure:*

1. Spray olive oil on each steak.

2. Sprinkle the steaks with seasoning, parsley and rosemary.

3. Grill steak over high heat. You can also cook in a broiler.

4. Serve hot with your favorite greens with light salad dressing on low-carb days. For high-carb days, you can add baked sweet potato or brown rice; and you can still have the veggies as side dish.

## Roasted Beef with Stir-Fry Veggies

*Ingredients:*

- 6 oz lean sirloin steak, boneless

- Olive oil in spray bottle

- 2 tsp low-sodium soy sauce

- ½ tsp cornstarch

- 1/8 ground ginger

- 1 tsp roasted garlic and bell pepper seasoning

- 1/3 cup assorted veggies (you can use snow peas, broccoli, and bell pepper strips)

- 1/3 cup water

*Note:* This recipe yields 2 portions, double the measurements if you need to make 4.

*Procedure:*

1. Cut the sirloin steak into 1/4 –inch strips.

2. In a mixing bowl, put the soy sauce, ginger, roasted garlic and bell pepper seasoning, cornstarch and water. Mix thoroughly and set aside.

3. Heat oil on medium to high setting in a non-stick pan. Add beef slices in small batches and cook each for about 5 minutes.

4. Spray more oil if needed.

5. When all the meat slices are done, cook the veggies in the same pan.

6. Serve with almonds or sliced avocado on your low-carb days or with brown rice on high-carb days.

### Low-Carb Blue Cheese Steak

*Ingredients:*

- 6 oz cube steak

- 1/3 cup blue cheese crumbles

- Olive oil in spray bottle

- Red onion, chopped

- ½ tbsp Salt and pepper

*Note:* This recipe serves 2, double or triple the portions if you need more.

*Procedure:*

1. Preheat broiler.

2. Heat a non-stick pan over medium heat and spray oil. Add the seasoned meat and cook on each side.

3. Line the broiler pan with foil and place the steak. Top meat with blue cheese and onion.

4. Broil until cheese melts.

5. Serve with steamed greens.

6. If you are making more portions and you want to freeze until you need them, after pan searing the meat, store in a zip-lock

plastic and put in the freezer. In a separate zip-lock bag, put onion and blue cheese and freeze as well. You can broil anytime meat is thawed or you can cook it in a microwave oven; just make sure to top the meat with blue cheese and onion.

### Sirloin Steak with Veggies

*Ingredients:*

- 6 oz lean sirloin steak, boneless

- Olive oil in spray bottle

- 1 cup green beans

- 1 medium tomato, chopped

- ¾ tsp garlic, minced

- Salt and pepper to taste

*Note:* This recipe can serve 1 to 2 persons, if you need to make more portions, adjust the measurements accordingly.

*Procedure:*

1. In a non-stick pan spray some oil and set stove to high heat. Add meat and cook on each side. Remove from pan and set aside.

2. Adjust heat to medium and in the same pan, add green beans and sauté for 3 minutes and then add garlic and cook for another one minute. Season with salt and pepper.

3. Add diced tomatoes and cook for a minute.

4. Cover pan and let the tomatoes become saucy, about 3 to 4 minutes.

5. Serve the meat with the vegetables on the side.

6. For low-carb days, add sliced avocado; and for high-carb days, serve with baked potato/ sweet potato or brown rice.

## Sweet Pork Tenderloin

*Ingredients:*

- 6 oz lean pork tenderloin
- 1 tbsp honey
- ½ tbsp vinegar
- ¼ tsp vanilla
- 1/8 tsp paprika
- A dash of ground mustard
- Salt and pepper to taste

*Note:* This makes 2 servings, adjust accordingly if you need more.

*Procedure:*

1. Combine honey and other flavorings in a zip-lock bag and mix well.
2. Add the pork tenderloin in the zip-lock bag and coat with the honey glaze all over.
3. Heat a non-stick pan over meat settings and cook pork tenderloin on each side.

4. Serve hot with a portion of pecans and vegetable salad on a low-carb day. On the other hand, you can serve it with baked sweet potato or brown rice and side salad for a high-carb day.

## Special Tenderloin with Herbs and Spices

*Ingredients:*

- 6 oz pork tenderloin, lean

- Olive oil in spray bottle

- ½ tsp paprika

- ¼ tsp dried thyme

- ¼ tsp salt

- 1/8 tsp black pepper

*Note:* The recipe is good for 2 persons so you can adjust measurements when needed.

*Procedure:*

1. In a mixing bowl, mix all the flavorings and spices. When thoroughly mixed, sprinkle over the pork tenderloins.

2. Spray oil on a non-stick pan and set to medium heat. Add the pork and cook on each side.

3. Serve with your choice of greens for a low-carb day or sweet potato for a high-carb day.

## Herbed Roast Pork with Garlic

*Ingredients:*

- 6 oz lean pork tenderloins

- Olive oil in spray bottle

- 2 tsp roasted garlic and herb seasoning

*Note:* This is good for 1 to 2 persons so if you need to feed more, adjust measurements.

*Procedure:*

1. Season pork with the roasted garlic and herb.

2. Spray oil on a non-stick pan and set to medium heat. Cook the pork tenderloin on each side.

3. This is perfect for a low-carb day when you serve with side salad with olive oil and balsamic dressing. If on a high-carb day, you can serve with steamed asparagus and brown rice.

### Grilled Chicken Wings

*Ingredients:*

- 4 pieces chicken wings

- Chicken spice mix seasoning

- Broccoli, asparagus, lettuce (or your choice of greens)

- Salsa

*Note:* This is good for 1 to 2 persons.

*Procedure:*

1. Preheat oven to 350°F.

2. Generously coat chicken wings with seasoning, making sure they are completely coated.

3. Insert chicken wings in the oven and cook until they are golden brown and crunchy.

4. Toss your choice of vegetables and top with salsa.

5. This is good for a low-carb day.

### Low-Carb Meatballs Barbecue

*Ingredients:*

- 1 lb ground pork, lean
- 1 tsp granulated sugar substitute
- 1 tsp paprika
- ½ tsp salt
- ¼ tsp black pepper
- ¼ tsp cayenne pepper
- ½ tsp ground cumin
- ¼ tsp celery salt
- 1 medium-sized egg
- ¼ cup almond flour
- 1 tbsp water

*For the BBQ Sauce*

- ¼ cup yellow mustard
- 2 tsp hot sauce
- 1 tbsp dried onion flakes

- 3 tbsp granulated sugar substitute

- 2 tbsp apple cider vinegar

- 2 tbsp ketchup

- Salt and pepper to taste

*Note:* This recipe makes 16 meatballs, 4 meatballs per serving.


*Procedure:*

1. First, mix all the barbecue sauce ingredients in a saucepan, stir until fully mixed and smooth. Over low heat, simmer sauce for about 8 minutes. Set aside.

2. In a mixing bowl, combine all the ingredients for the meatballs and mix. Form into medium-sized balls, this will give you 16 pieces.

3. In a non-stick skillet, fry meatballs over medium heat. Cooking time is 3 to 4 minutes on each side.

4. Toss the cooked meatballs into the barbecue sauce. Once meatballs are fully coated, spread them on a baking dish lined with parchment paper. Broil for about 2 to 3 minutes.

5. Serve with coleslaw or your favorite greens.

## Low-Carb Roasted Turkey

*Ingredients:*

- 1 whole turkey
- 1 tbsp vegetable oil
- 1 tsp Italian seasoning
- Salt and pepper

*Note:* This yields at least 18 servings.

*Procedure:*

1. Preheat your outdoor grill to get medium to high heat.

2. Prepare the turkey. After washing it clean, pat to dry. Turn the wings back so the neck skin is held in place. Turn the legs to a tucked position.

3. Brush turkey skin with oil. Season both inside and out with the Italian seasoning, salt and pepper.

4. Position the turkey, with the breast side up, on the metal grate inside a large roasting pan. Place the pan on the prepared grill.

5. Cooking time is 2 to 3 hours.

6. Remove from the grill and let it stand for about 15 minutes before carving the turkey.

7.  Serve with your favorite greens.

### Delicious Salmon Fillet with Herbs and Spices

*Ingredients:*

- 4 pieces salmon fillet, no bones and skin
- ½ cup melted unsalted butter
- 2 tbsp ground paprika
- 1 tbsp ground cayenne pepper
- 1 tbsp onion powder
- 2 tsp salt
- ½ tsp ground white pepper
- ½ tsp ground black pepper
- ¼ tsp dried thyme
- ¼ tsp dried basil
- ¼ tsp dried oregano

*Note:* This recipe yields 4 servings.

*Procedure:*

1. In a mixing bowl, mix the spices: paprika, cayenne pepper, salt, onion powder, white and black pepper, basil, thyme and oregano.

2. Brush each salmon fillet with ¼ of the butter and evenly sprinkle with the mixed spices.

3. Drizzle on each side with half of the remaining butter.

4. Heat a large skillet to high and cook salmon, with the butter side down, until crust is blackened; this will take about 2 to 5 minutes.

5. Turn the fillet and drizzle with the last remaining butter.

6. Continue cooking until crust is blackened. It is ready when fish is flaked when you poke with a fork.

### Spicy Pork Tenderloin

*Ingredients:*

- 6 oz pork tenderloin
- 1 tsp butter
- Olive oil in spray bottle
- ½ tsp paprika
- ¼ dried oregano
- ½ tsp garlic powder
- ½ tsp ground cumin
- ¾ tsp salt
- 1/8 tsp fennel seeds
- A dash of ground cayenne pepper
- ¼ cup chicken broth

*Note:* This recipe makes 2 servings.

*Procedure:*

1. In a small mixing bowl, combine all the herbs and spices.
2. Brush half of the spice on one side of the tenderloin.

3. Set non-stick pan to medium heat and add the pork, with the spiced side down. While pork is cooking in that position, sprinkle the rest of the spices on top.

4. Cook on each side until browned.

5. Remove from pan and keep the pork warm.

6. On the same pan, add butter and whisk all the browned bits and spices left in the pan. Turn the heat to medium-high and add the chicken broth. Continue whisking until sauce is reduced by half.

7. Place the pork on a serving plate and drizzle the sauce on top.

8. Serve with your potato salad or baked potato for a high-carb day or your favorite greens for a low-carb day.

### *Easy Garlic and Herb Shrimp Salad*

*Ingredients:*

- 25 pieces large shrimps, peeled and deveined

- Olive oil in a spray bottle

- 2 tsp roasted garlic and herb seasoning

- Raw baby spinach

*Note:* This makes 2 servings.

*Procedure:*

1. Thoroughly season shrimp with roasted garlic and herb mix.

2. Spray oil on a non-stick pan and set to medium heat.

3. Cook shrimp.

4. Serve immediately over a bed of baby spinach. You can toss spinach with balsamic vinegar and olive oil before adding the shrimp.

### Perfect Salmon Fillet

*Ingredients:*

- 8 oz salmon fillet

- ½ tbsp butter

- 1 tbsp Cajun seasoning

- 1 tsp minced garlic

- 2 tbsp balsamic vinegar

- 2 lemon wedges

*Note:* Makes 2 servings. Add portions to make more.

*Procedure:*

1. Heat a non-stick pan set at medium heat. Melt butter and add salmon. Cook on each side but you have to be careful because salmon cooks rather quickly. If salmon is overcooked, it becomes dry.

2. Remove fish from pan and keep warm.

3. On the same pan, add in the rest of the butter, then add garlic and Cajun seasoning.

4. Cook for about 2 minutes before adding the balsamic vinegar. Simmer for another 2 minutes, with continuous stirring.

5. Put back the salmon to the pan and finish the cooking process.

6. Place the fillet on a serving plate and garnish with lemon wedges.

7. Serve with steamed asparagus or baby spinach if you are on a low-carb day. When you are on a high-carb day, add brown rice.

# Chapter 5: You can be Healthy

The recipes in this book are easy to understand and prepare, so you don't have to worry if you are not a cooking-pro because the recipes have been given to you in a step-by-step manner. When you cook your own food, it is easier to track what you are eating and you don't need to worry if you are eating right and healthy. Each of the recipes are based on the basic foundation which includes the low-carb and high-carb variations.

The recipes are still customizable. You have a lot of endless possibilities in creating delicious and healthy meals.

Losing weight is not just about eating healthy foods but also eating the right portions. While there are a lot of applications that you can download to help you keep track of the amount of calories that you eat, it is still important that you know how portioning works.

*Hand Portioning*

Did you know that your hands are the best guide in determining how much portion you can eat?

- For proteins, the best portion is just about the size and thickness of your palm.

- For carbohydrates, the perfect portion is the size of your clenched fist.

- Take the size of your two clenched fists that is the ideal portion for the vegetables. However, you can have as many veggies as you want, there is no limitation.

- The size of your thumb starting from the base up is the amount of fat you can have daily.

- The portion for the condiments, sauces, and dressings should not be larger than the size of your index finger and middle finger starting from the base up.

*What you can Include in Your Diet*

Aside from the recipes above, you will have examples of carb-cycling foods that you are allowed to have:

## Protein:

### Beef

- Cube steak – 2.5 oz

- Low sodium roast beef - 3 oz

- Extra lean sirloin steak – 2 oz

- Lean flank steak – 2.5 oz

- Venison – 2 oz

### Dairy

- Cottage cheese ½ cup

- Egg whites – 4 whites

- Egg substitutes – 1 cup

- Plain Greek yogurt -3/4 cup

  *Lean Ground Meats*

- Extra lean ground beef – 2 oz

- Ground chicken breast – 4 oz

- Ground turkey – 3 oz

### Poultry

- Duck breast – 2 oz

- Skinless chicken thigh – 3 oz

- Skinless chicken breast – 3.5 oz

  *Powdered*

- Whey, soy, hemp, rice – 1 scoop

### Fish

- Salmon fillet – 2 oz

- Sardines – 52 g (4 sardines)

- Canned tuna – 3 oz

- Tuna fillet – 3 oz

- White fish – 2.5 oz

### Shellfish

- Raw clams – 5 oz

- Shrimp/lobster – 4 oz

*Vegetable Protein*

- Tempeh – 2 oz

- Tofu – 4 oz

*White Meat*

- Pork tenderloin – 2.5 oz


## Carbohydrates:


### Bread

- Corn tortillas – 1 ½ servings

- Bread – 1 slice

- English muffin – ½ piece


### Cereal

- Low-fat granola – ½ cup

- Old-fashioned oatmeal (cooked) – ¾ cup

### Grains

- Buckwheat, Bran, Barley, Brown Rice – ½ cup

- Oats (steel-cut, cooked) – 2/3 cup

- Popcorn (no oil) – 3 cups

- Quinoa – ½ cup

- Wild rice – ½ cup

### Legumes

- Beans – ½ cup

- Lentils – ½ cup

- Soybeans – ¼ cup

- Soy nuts - 3 tbsp

### Pasta

- Brown rice pasta – ½ cup

- Couscous – ½ cup

- Whole grain – ½ cup

### Root Vegetables

- Carrots – 2 cups

- Potatoes – ¾ cup

- Beets – 1 ½ cups

- Yams and sweet potatoes – 2/3 cup


### Starchy Vegetables

- Peas – 1 cup

- Corn - 2/3 cup

**Fruits:**

### Fresh

- Apricots – 6 pieces

- Banana – 1 piece

- Apples – 1 ½

- Berries, like blueberries, cherries, and strawberries – 1 ½ cups

- Grapes – 1 ½ cups

- Oranges – 1 piece

- Melons – 1 ½ cups

- Mangoes – 1 cup

- Lemons and limes – 5 pieces

- Papayas – 2 cups

- Plums – 3 ½ pieces

- Pineapple – ½ cup

- Peaches – 2 large pieces

- Pears – 1 piece

- Grapefruit – 1 piece

- Kiwi – 4 pieces

## Vegetables:

- Asparagus – 3 ½ cups
- Artichokes – 2 pieces, medium-sized
- Broccoli – 4 cups
- Brussels sprouts – 2 ½ cups
- Bok Choy – 1 head
- Cabbage – 4 cups
- Chard – 10 leaves
- Celery – 5 cups
- Cauliflower – 4 cups
- Collard greens – 10 cups
- Eggplant – 5 cups
- Garlic – 20 cloves
- Fennel – 4 cups
- Green beans – 75 pieces
- Kale – 3 cups
- Mushrooms – 20 large pieces
- Leeks – 2 pieces
- Okra – 2 pieces medium-sized
- Radish – 5 cups

- Scallions – 10 cups

- Snow peas – 70 pods

- Parsley – 4 cups

- Spinach – 10 cups

- Tomatoes – 6 ½ pieces, medium-sized

- Turnips – 2 large pieces

- Zucchini – 2 large pieces

## *Fats:*

*Dairy:*

- Cream cheese – 2 tbsp

- Egg yolk – 2

- Whip cream – 2 tbsp

- Mozzarella – 1 oz

- Parmesan – 1 oz

- Romano – 1 oz

### Nuts and Seeds:

- Almonds – 1 ½ tbsp

- Peanut butter – 1 tbsp

- Pecans – 1 ½ tbsp

- Sesame seeds – 2 tbsp

- Sunflower seeds – 1 ½ tbsp


### Beverages:

- Black coffee – unlimited

- Unsweetened soy milk – 1 ¼ cup

- Tea (herbal, green) – unlimited

- Water – unlimited

- Tomato juice – 2 ½ cups

Now that you have been given easy to follow and prepare carb cycling food recipes, you don't have any excuse to lose weight. Don't worry if you cannot cook all the time because of work and household chores, you can bulk-prepare your foods and store in the fridge. You can easily reheat and eat!

# Conclusion

I'd like to thank you and congratulate you for transiting my lines from start to finish.

I hope this book was able to help you to lose weight and change your life for the better.

The next step is to take the things that you have learned to heart and try cooking the recipes in this book. Share this with your family and friends so they can get the life they want too.

It's time for you to transcend the written word and keep on fighting for what you want in life. Go out there and fight for what is yours!

I wish you the best of luck!

To your success,

*John Web*

Made in the USA
Lexington, KY
26 June 2019